Fantastic
Fore
play

Quarto.com

© 2024 Quarto Publishing Group
USA Inc.
Text © 2013, 2024 Jessica O'Reilly, Ph.D.

First Published in 2024 by Fair Winds
Press, an imprint of The Quarto Group,
100 Cummings Center, Suite 265-D,
Beverly, MA 01915, USA.
T (978) 282-9590 F (978) 283-2742

Fair Winds Press titles are also available
at discount for retail, wholesale,
promotional, and bulk purchase.
For details, contact the Special Sales
Manager by email at specialsales@
quarto.com or by mail at The Quarto
Group, Attn: Special Sales Manager, 100
Cummings Center, Suite 265-D, Beverly,
MA 01915, USA.

28 27 26 25 24   1 2 3 4 5

ISBN: 978-0-7603-9253-9

Digital edition published in 2024
eISBN: 978-0-7603-9254-6

Library of Congress Control Number
available.

Compiled and edited by Jill Hamilton
Design and layout: Burge Agency
Illustration: Sandra Alutyte

Printed in Hong Kong

The information in this book is for
educational purposes only. Any type of
sexual activity should be consensual.

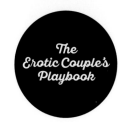

The Erotic Couple's Playbook

Fantastic
Fore
play

QUIVER

Contents

Part 1
Pussy Play

11

Part 2
Cock Games

Introduction

"Foreplay" used to mean a little boob play before the real sex, i.e. penetration, started. But now couples of all kinds know that foreplay—mutual masturbation, oral sex, toys—is just as sexy, intimate, and orgasmic as penetration. If not more so. Foreplay includes everything from whatever gets you in the mood to moves that get you closer to orgasm. Some of the "foreplay" might get you so close to coming that *omgomg* you're already there. And that is all good.

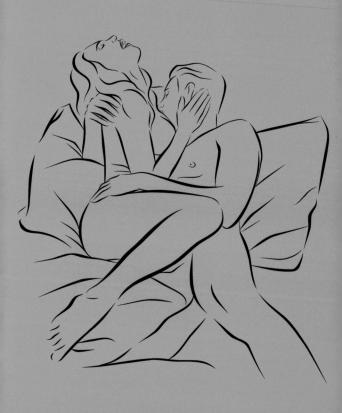

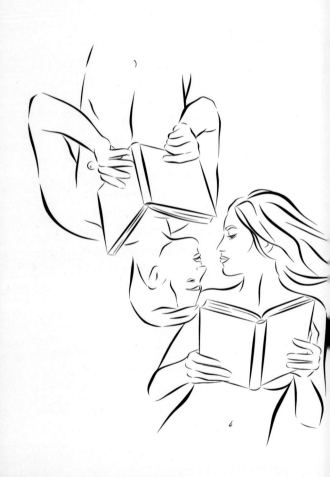

How to Use This Book

Here's a bunch of ideas. Like a big-ass Cheesecake Factory menu, you might not like everything. Do the ones that sound fun. Or be brave and try some that sound trippy—you might find a new thing you're into. (If something sounds *bad*, then for F's sake, don't do it. Rip the page out. That one is dead to you.) The idea is to get you both panting, wet/hard, and desperate for each other. When one of you feels like they'll completely lose it if the other one doesn't touch you, slide inside of you, fire up that toy, etc… *this very second*… you're doing foreplay right.

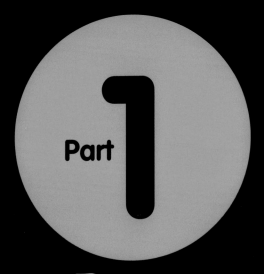

Part **1**

Pussy
Play

Vulvas, Vaginas, and Clits, Oh My!

1. **Vulva**: All the parts on the outside of a woman's genitals, including the lips, clitoris, mons, vaginal opening, and urethral opening. Sometimes when people say "vagina" they mean "vulva."

2. **Labia majora**: The large fleshy lips on either side of the inner labia which may be covered in pubic hair.

3. **Labia minora**: Hairless lips that range in color from light pink to a dark brownish black and in size from small to prominent. They're sensitive and swell when aroused.

4. **Mons or Venus mound**: The soft area of fatty tissue above the pubic bone which may be covered in hair.

5. **Clitoris**: Most people think of the clitoris as the tip but it's actually an extensive structure of erectile tissue, both internal and external, including a head, hood, shaft, bulbs, and legs. It swells when aroused and is designed solely for pleasure.

6. **Clitoral head**: This highly sensitive tip is located at the top of the vulva where the inner lips meet. Most people need some sort of clitoral stimulation—direct or indirect, depending on owner—to reach orgasm.

7. **Clitoral hood**: A bit of foreskin that covers and protects the clitoral head. It may retract when the clitoral head swells.

8. **Clitoral shaft**: Attached to the clitoral head, when erect it wraps around the vagina on the inside of the body.

9. **Clitoral legs**: Two long internal legs that form a V-shape around the vaginal walls and urethra.

10. **Clitoral bulbs**: Located internally beneath the outer labia, these internal bulbs swell with arousal and cause the rhythmic contractions during orgasms.

11. **Vagina**: This tubelike canal is composed of mucous membranes and enclosed by elastic tissue and muscles. Vaginas can be penetrated with toys, a penis, or fingers. Some people like rhythmic pressure against the top wall of the vagina, an area some people call the G-spot but is now considered part of the internal clitoris.

12. **Urethral opening**: The tiny hole below the clitoris where urine and ejaculate come out.

13. **Anus**: A.K.A., the butt hole. As it is filled with sensitive nerve endings, many people like anal stimulation with a finger, the mouth, toys, or penetration. (Note: The anus and rectum are not self-lubricating, so with any anal play, make sure to use a lot of lube and go slowly.)

14. **Perineum**: The smooth area of skin, also called the taint, between the lower vulva and the anus. Some people like a tongue, a vibrator, or a finger pressed against it.

The Vulva and
Surrounding Areas

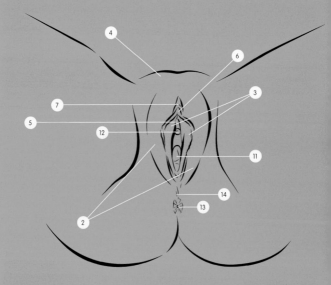

Breathing You In

01

Explore your partner's body with nothing but your warm breath. Have them lie on their stomach. Bring your lips to their foot and breathe gently on their toes. Work your way very slowly up the outside of their legs, over their calf, knee, and thigh, then back down the center of their leg. Spread their legs a bit, then take your time brushing your lips up their inner leg, pausing to breathe gently on their vulva (not actually *in* the vagina, that's unsafe). Repeat with the other leg the same love and they will be panting for you!

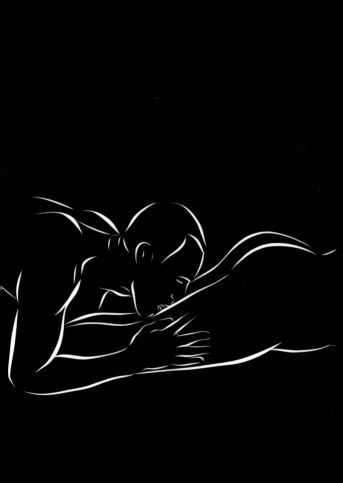

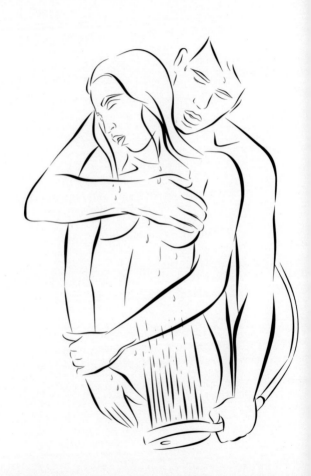

Worked Into a Lather

02

Use the privacy of a steamy shower to soap each other up. Take your time, lathering each part and describing just what ravishment awaits your partner after you dry them off. Make soapy circles around their nipples, or slide your fingers between their legs and linger a bit. If it turns into a full-on handie, oral, or penetration, completely valid. No rules in the shower, except hold on to something sturdy to avoid an embarrassing slip and fall.

Tell Me a Story

03

Everyone has that one fantasy that sends them over the edge every time. Harness the prodigious power of that fantasy by having your partner lie face down with their hips propped up on a pillow or two. Kneel behind them and ask them to tell you that fantasy while you kiss and stroke their vulva, thighs, and clit. Make them feel safe enough to tell you their *real* favorite fantasy, the one that's kind of pervy and shameful—but so very hot. (Facing away helps with fantasy-sharing bravery since there's no eye contact.)

Urge them deeper with encouraging words while plying them with your fingers and mouth. So worth it for both of you. Few things are hotter than hearing your partner have to stop telling the story because they're so turned on they can barely keep it together.

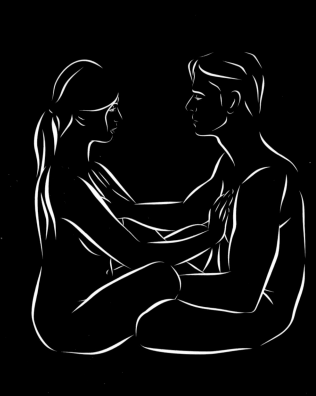

Yab Yummmm

04

Go deep with the intimacy by trying some beginner tantra in the Yab Yum position. Sit facing each other, cross-legged, with one person's legs wrapped around the other's hips. Put one hand on each other's chest and gaze into each other's eyes. (If that's waaaaay too much lookin', touch your foreheads together for 100% less eye contact.) Breath in sync and behold how connected you feel. If you want to move into penetration, try grinding instead of thrusting.

Pussy Pocket

Have them lie on their belly. Fill your hand with lube and from behind, slide your hand under their hips and cup your hand against their vulva. You can rub with your whole hand up and down over their outer lips, curl your hands to create a pulsing sensation or open and close your fingers over their lips. If they start wildly humping your hand, that's perfect. Keep doing exactly what you're doing. Do. Not. Stop.

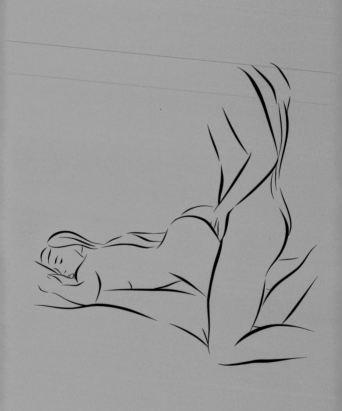

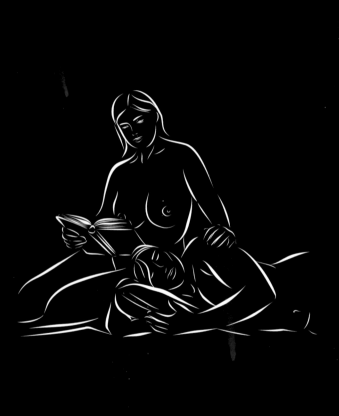

Erotica City

06

Read them their choice of erotica while lightly cupping their pussy. Start slowly and gently, pressing and pulsing on their outer lips. Match your intensity to the pace of the story. When the story gets to the good parts, slide your fingers between their lips to increase the stimulation. (For what it's worth, this is a judgement-free zone. Whatever kind of erotica you're into, go for it!)

Deep V Diving

07

If you don't know what your partner likes, get on down there and figure it out. Explore their vulva, clitoris, and vagina with your mouth and fingers. Go ahead and ask your partner what they like as you touch each part: the labia, the clitoral head, the mons, etc. (see glossary on page 12 for more details). Ask them to rank each touch from 1 to 10. The goal here isn't orgasm, it's collecting valuable intel for the future.

The Ultimate Finger F*ck

08

The key to a stellar finger f*ck is going slowly to make them want more. Start with two fingers astride their clit. With your other hand, make slow circles around the entrance to their vagina. Slide a finger in about a centimeter. Thrust, just to that point, about 10 times, asking them to squeeze around you. Repeat, going deeper until your finger is rubbing the upper wall of the vagina, while you continue to rub their clit.

Thigh Highs

09

Blindfold your partner—with permission, obviously—to make it easier for them to focus on your every touch. (Blindfolds are good like that.) Lie your partner on their back and spread their legs. Kiss and lick your way up their thighs, telling them how hot they look. Drizzle warm lube onto their inner thighs and belly and massage your way up and around their vulva without actually touching it. If/when they beg, go ahead and touch.

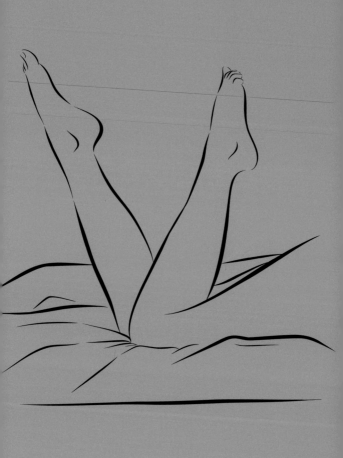

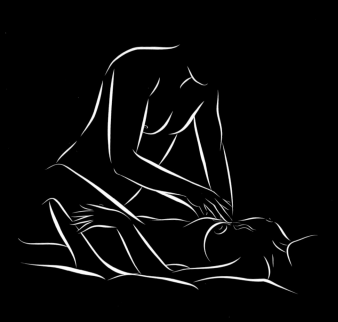

Lube Job

10

Fill a glass with warm water and stick a bottle of lube in there for 10 to 15 minutes to warm it. Use your fingers to paint lube all over your partner's body. Paint their nipples, belly, and up their inner thighs. Tease them by painting around their vulva—not touching it—until they start moaning and/or pressing their hips up for more. Then and only then, spread their lips and paint over their vulva, clit, and perineum.

Open and Shut

11

People can rub their own vulvas just fine, BUT they can't do this particular move by themselves. And that, my friend, is how to make yourself indispensable. Sit your partner down at the edge of the bed, with their knees apart. Kneel on the floor between their legs, and make a V with your lubed fingers on either side of their clit. Slide your hand down, gently closing your middle and index finger over their inner lips.

Then slide your hand back up, scissoring your fingers back open at your approach their clit. Repeat in a smooth motion. You can reverse it by starting with the open V fingers at the bottom of their vulva then closing your fingers as you move up or, if you're feeling advanced, using two hands, one doing each variation.

It's a Vibe

12

Early vibrators were marketed as for "massage," but TBH, they were mostly used for wanking. Use one for both purposes by using a vibrator to combine a massage with a happy ending. Have your partner lie face down (a million extra bonus points if you drape them in a blanket straight from the dryer). Run the vibrator over their arms, back, shoulders, down their legs, up their upper thighs and butt, until they start spreading their legs for more. When they're ready, start at the sides of the vulva, running it over the outer lips and see how much stimulation they can handle.

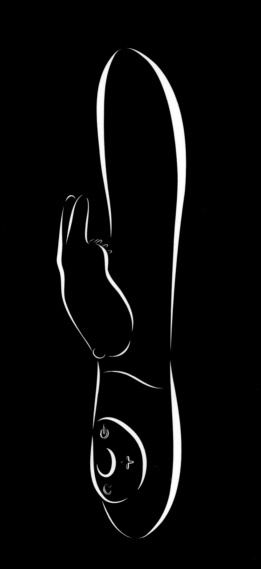

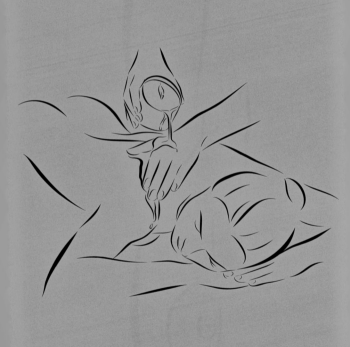

Make Them Melt

13

Light a candle that melts into massage oil and give your partner a long, luxurious massage. (PSA: Do NOT use a regular candle—the wax gets way too hot.) Take your time giving an actual good massage, not the perfunctory kind that means "I want to get laid." Work your way towards their butt and thighs, teasing around their vulva. If they arch their back for more of you, switch to regular lube before going in.

I Declare a Thumb War

Thumbs don't have a rep of being a particularly sexy body part, but when called into duty, they can be surprisingly useful. There are several ways to use those sexy, sexy opposable thumbs:

1. Press your two thumbs of either side of your partner's clit, stroking outward or up and down as you suck gently on their clit.

2. Slide your lubed thumb inside your partner's vagina, pressing against the upper wall. Slide it back out, curling it upward in a scooping motion to stroke the clit. Keep this motion going and use your other thumb to press and slide against the lower wall of the vagina.

3. Put your thumbs on either side of the clit, pressing them together to make the clitoral head jut out a bit. Make slow circles around their clit with your tongue or flatten your tongue and swipe your tongue side to side.

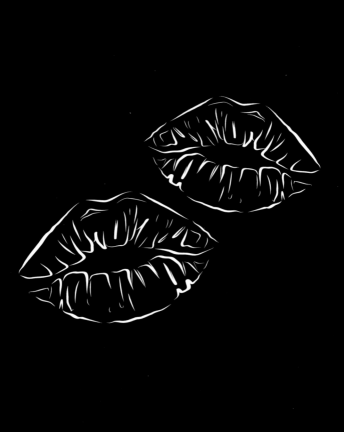

Kiss and Tell

15

If your partner's love language is "words of affirmation," here's your new go-to move. Explore them with your mouth and hands, and as you go, describe what you're seeing and how much you love it, saying things like "I can't get enough of you," "You're making me so hard/wet," or "You are so fucking sexy." Impossible to go too hard here, but adjust the dirtiness of your words according to taste.

Tongue-Tied

16

Restraints are a great way to play around with power dynamics, but they can also help the restrainee fully relax into the experience. Use hand cuffs or DIY it with ties or scarves, and bind your partner's wrists together behind their head. Use just your tongue to explore their entire body, keeping a safe word at the ready in case it gets too intense. (As with any BDSM play, trust, communication, and aftercare are non-negotiable.)

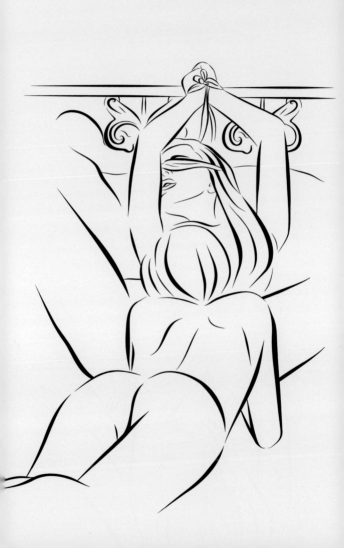

Hump Day

17

For people whose first sexual experience was humping a pillow, their hand, or an innocent teddy bear, give them the kind of stimulation that really does it for them. Have them straddle a pillow with your well-lubed hand atop the pillow and your palm facing up so they can rock back and forth against your palm and fingers. For extra oomph, put a powerful wand vibrator under your hand to ply them with your Incredible Vibrating Hand.

I'm Sooo Close

18

The head of the clitoris is very sensitive,
sometimes so sensitive that direct touch
is just way too much. If that's the kind of
clit you're working with, you're gonna
have to approach it gently. It still wants
stimulation, but not *on* the clit—try *near*
the clit for a more diffuse sensation.
Use gentle circles around the clit with
a wet finger, tapping on the sides of
the clit, and/or rubbing two fingers on
either side.

Get on Their Good Side

Most people have an area of their clit that's most sensitive. It's generally a tiny spot on the part of their clitoral shaft, at about 10 o'clock or 2 o'clock depending on if they're a "rightie" or "leftie." For some people, stimulating this spot is crucial for getting to orgasm. Some people like very focused attention to the spot, so use the tip of your tongue, your fingertip, or a buzzy vibrator (there are vibrators with a pointed tip for just this purpose). For other people, that's too intense, so rub against it with your flat tongue, the side of your finger, or just press and hold a vibrator with low, rumbly vibes on the spot. Figure out which your partner likes and act accordingly. It might seem like you're barely doing anything, but by focusing on just that one spot, you can give your partner one hell of an orgasm.

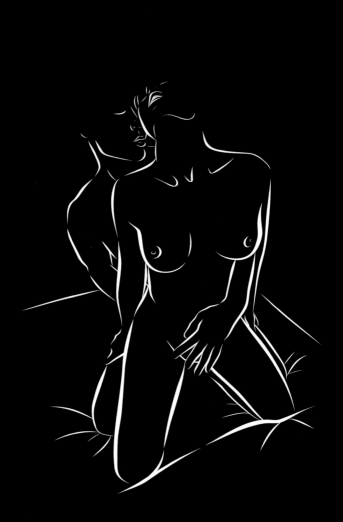

Double Hand Job

20

As a prelude to standing penetrative sex, or as the sex itself, get your hands lubed up. (Lubing up body parts is pretty much always a stellar idea, sex-wise.) Stand beside your partner, using one hand to slide up and down their butt crack and the other to slide up their vulva. Use a sweeping upstroke or stroke up and down. Caveat: Don't switch your hands though—what happens at the butt needs to stay at the butt.

Here, Kitty Kitty

To create optimal conditions for (possible) squirting, stimulate the area formerly known as the G-spot. Use a hand or a toy on their clit, then slide a finger of the other hand into their vagina to stroke the upper wall, just an inch or two in. You can curl your finger up in the "come hither" gesture, tap or just press firmly. If no squirting happens, *totally* normal, most people don't. Either way, this move still feels amazing.

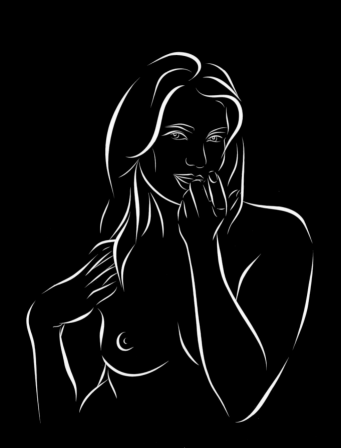

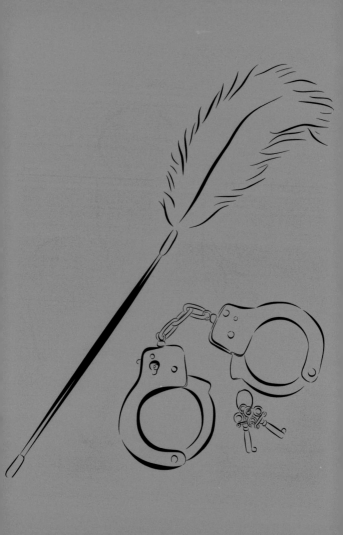

Choose Your Weapon(s)

22

Create anticipation for a BDSM session by putting out an array of gear like handcuffs, blindfold, feather teaser, and/or a paddle. Ask them to choose their punishment. Take your time getting each piece of equipment out, dramatically strapping them on or doing a test smack on their bum. Whisper something sexy as you tie on their blindfold or kiss the palms of their hands as you cuff their wrists. (Hugely important BDSM caveat: This is all consensual. Have a safe word, discuss the scene beforehand, stop immediately if someone's uncomfortable, and practice good aftercare.)

Off-and-On Relationship

Edging is about getting your partner super close to orgasm then pulling back. The idea is torquing their arousal until all they can think about is finally, FINALLY getting that orgasm. Which you will give them. . . eventually. It'll be worth it too because orgasms after an edging session can feel deeper, stronger, and eminently satisfying. Plus, edging adds a whole element of power play. For the edgee, it can be an intense experience to surrender to another person. For the edger, it's just as powerful to take someone to that place of surrender. Here's how to get there.

Press a vibrator against your partner's vulva, then move it away for a moment. Repeat with the pattern of stimulation, taking them to the point of orgasm, but stopping *just* before. When they look like they're gonna kill you if you don't keep the vibe pressed against them, keep it there. Or you'll be sorry.

The Suck 'N Tuck

24

Using two toys at once is at least twice as good. For the ultimate toy synergy, hold a suction vibrator toy gently over your partner's clit. You don't need to move it around—these toys have it all figured out, so just hold it there. As they get more turned on, bust out a vibrating G-spot toy and slide it inside them, pressing it against the upper wall of their vagina. Fire it up, and hold on!

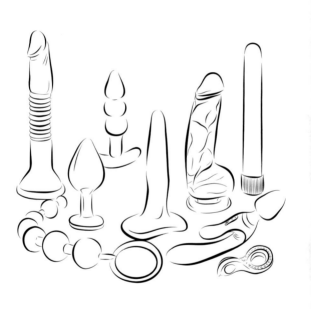

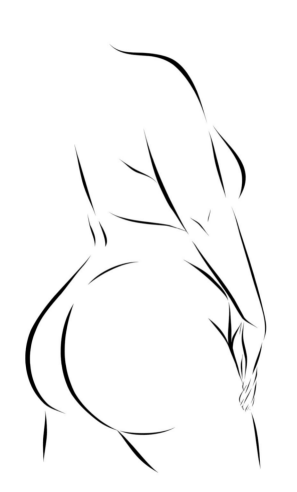

Butter Up

25

Butt stuff should always happen when the butt's owner is already turned on. Make sure your partner is ready by treating them to some of your finest oral sex. Have a well-lubed butt plug at hand. (Butts are not self-lubricating, so lube the hell out of everything.) As you work on their vulva with your mouth, slowly slide a vibrating plug around your partner's butt hole, then all the way into their butt and let it rumble away.

The Full Power

26

Wand vibrators are the jackhammer of sex toys. No subtlety, just full-on power. Harness that power for good by having your partner lie on top of it and firing that thing up. While they ride the waves of rumbling vibrations, you can slide a finger or dildo inside them (either hole, y'all's choice) or just rub their ass in support. If the vibrations feel too hardcore (valid), use a pillow or rolled up t-shirts as a buffer.

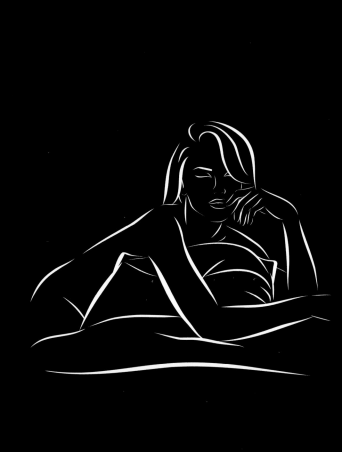

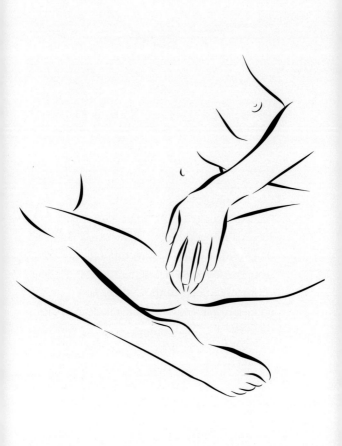

The MMMMMM

27

Get maximum hand-to-vulva contact by lubing your hand and making an M with your fingers. Press your thumb and index finger together and your pinkie and ring finger together. Slowly slide your hand down, pressing their clit with your middle finger and gently squeezing their inner lips. Reverse the move, sliding your hand back up. You can stick with the up and down motion, rub in wide circles, or go side-to-side.

Fifth Base

28

If grown-ups still used the sexual base system, fifth base would be butt stuff. Try sliding a finger in your partner's bum and a thumb in their vagina. Pinch them together and thrust with your hand, while rubbing their vulva with a hand or toy. If it's a first butt experience, make sure you go very slowly. Use a literal buttload of lube and start by teasing around their butt hole, making sure they're extremely turned on before any penetration.

The Spanking Machine

29

Bend them over a counter, spread their legs apart and use a wand vibrator on their vulva. Alternate with sharp smacks on their butt, using your hand or a paddle. Don't follow a particular pattern. Keep your partner on edge, awaiting your next move. Each sensation heightens the other. (Reminder, again: This is all consensual. Have a safe word, discuss the scene beforehand, stop immediately if someone's uncomfortable, and practice good aftercare.)

The Triple Play

30

For foreplay that's less like a warm-up and more like "this is actually sex that's happening," get your partner's butt, vagina, and clit all fired up at once. Having all three of them filled and/or rubbed at the same time is pretty epic. (As with all sex things, getting consent is crucial before any anal play. No one likes surprise butt stuff.) If you want to go old-school, use a combo of fingers. Stick a thumb into their butt, the other thumb into their vagina and your fingers on their vulva. Or mimic double penetration with a dildo in each hole and your mouth on their vulva. Or opt for any mix of hands, toys, and mouth. Dildo + butt plug + mouth! A two-pronged vibrating toy that goes into the vagina and butt + your fingers rubbing their clit. Anything's possible—it's up to you, my friend.

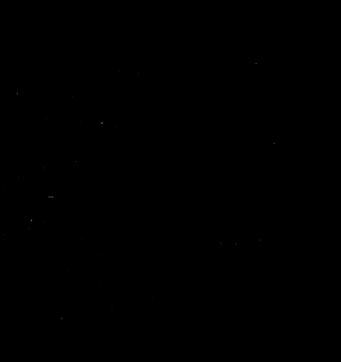

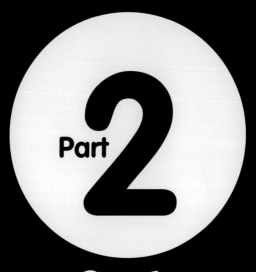

Part 2

Cock Games

A Cock-and-Balls Story: An Anatomical Glossary

1. **Head**: Also known as the tip or the glans, this is the bulbous part at the end of the shaft and is the most sensitive part of the penis. It also contains the opening to the urethra, the small hole where pre-ejaculate (pre-cum), semen, and urine come out.

2. **Shaft**: The shaft is the main part of the penis between the head and where it connects to the body. It looks like a tube and is made of spongey tissue that expands during erections.

3. **Corona**: This is the flared ridge surrounding the base of the head. It responds to touch and swells during arousal.

4. **Frenulum**: The little piece of connective tissue on the underside of the penis at the top of the shaft and base of the head. It's very sensitive to direct stimulation.

5. **Foreskin**: The protective layer of skin that covers the head of the penis. If a person has been circumcised, the foreskin has been removed and the head is more visible. If the person is uncircumcised, the head is partially covered with the foreskin. Uncircumcised people often have more sensitivity in their penis.

6. **Testicles**: Commonly known as balls, they're inside the scrotal sac and produce sperm cells. They're extremely sensitive to pain. They retract closer to the body via a muscle called the cremaster when a person is cold or nearing orgasm.

7. **Scrotum**: Also known as the ball sack, this is the soft skin sac that contain the testicles. Some people like gentle touches, tugs, and licks on the scrotum.

8. **Perineum**: A.K.A., the taint, this is the sensitive space between the anus and the base of the scrotum. Some people like a tongue, a vibrator, or a finger pressed against it.

9. **Prostate**: Also called the P-spot, the prostate is an internal walnut-shaped gland. It can be accessed by pressing against the upper wall of the rectum with hand or toy. Stimulating it can give some people a "P-gasm," which can feel deeper and produce more ejaculate.

10. **Anus**: A.K.A., the butt hole. It has lots of sensitive nerve endings, and many people like anal stimulation with a finger, the mouth, toys, or penetration. (Note: The anus and rectum are not self-lubricating, so with any anal play, make sure to use a lot of lube and go slowly.)

The Penis and Surrounding Areas

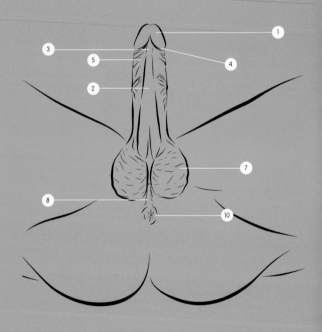

Naked Day

01

Spend a weekend day at home completely naked (or it that's a little *too* naked for you, just wearing a shirt à la Winnie the Pooh). Tell your partner they can't have you until later that night. Go about your regular business, letting them imagine what's coming later. It's totally fair to tease your partner throughout the day with long kisses while you press against them, an occasional squeeze on the butt, or by applying lotion to yourself more often than necessary.

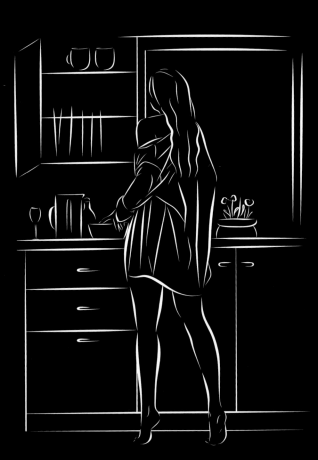

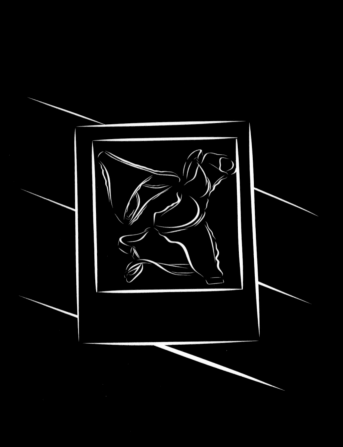

The AV Club

02

Right before they're going to see you, slip away to your room and send your partner a series of photos and recordings, letting them know exactly what's going on in there. Send a photo of your panties on the floor by your ankles, a slo-mo video of lube dripping onto your fingers, a series of sexts telling them what you're doing, and an audio-only video of your moans as you slide your hand between your legs.

We Can't

Recreate your insanely hot first sexual experience together with an old school make out session. Stay fully clothed for accuracy, with desperate dry humping against each other, hot breaths against zippers, and the general idea that what you're doing is probably wrong, so very, very wrong. Spend lots of time kissing, nibbling along your partner's jaw line, pressing your lips to their neck, and sucking gently on their earlobes. Keep your clothes on as long as possible, revealing each new body part like it's a present, to recreate the feeling of "OMG, I'm touching a boob!" Then take your time before unveiling the next part. Before taking off your underwear, for example, breathe hotly against the fabric, nibble with your lips around outline of their penis, dip your tongue into their underwear to just lick the head of the penis, then take their whole head in your mouth.

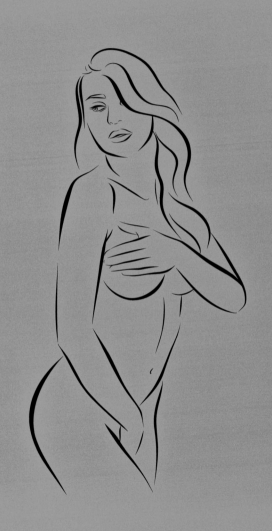

Watch and Learn

04

Let your partner watch as you touch yourself. The rule is that they can't touch you—at least not yet—only watch as you ravish yourself. You *could* be a little porno about it and exaggerate everything, BUT it's way hotter if you touch yourself like you really do when you're alone. You'll get the stimulation that actually does it for you, but even better, you're giving them a private lesson on exactly how to touch you.

Blindfolded Stripping

What good is stripping if your partner can't see you? Oh, so very good. Sit them down, blindfolding them. Explain in detail what you're doing as you remove each piece of clothing (i.e. "I'm unhooking my bra and squeezing my boob a little for you.") As you go, tease them by brushing a nipple across their cheeks, touching your panties to their lips, and pressing their hand between your legs to feel you.

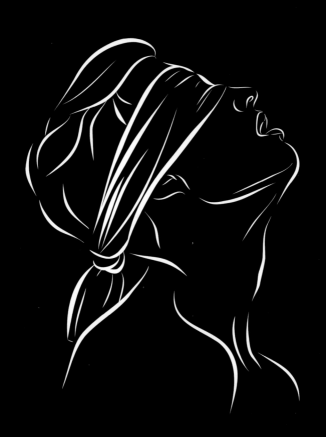

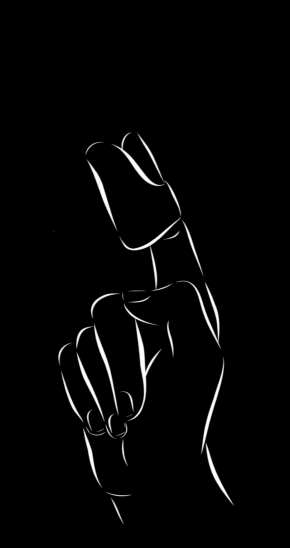

Magic Fingers

06

Show your partner just how fun a good vibe can be by using your mouth and vibe to explore their body. A simple finger vibe is good for first-timers because its vibrations are not too intense. Start by using the vibe to draw circles around their nipples. Kiss your way down their belly then circle the vibe around, but not on, their penis. Press it into their upper thighs, their pubic hair, and over their perineum. If they like it and give you the go-ahead, try sliding the vibe up the underside of their penis, holding it on the perineum while you stroke their shaft or suck their penis.

Air Head

07

If y'all can stand a little teasing (yes,
please!), bust out some Air Head. This
is all about making your partner unable
to think of anything besides how much
they want your mouth on them. Start by
kissing your way up their thighs then
pausing between their legs. Lick your
lips and gaze lasciviously at their cock.
Wrap your fingers around the base of
their shaft and put your mouth around

their cock without making contact. Breathe your warm breath onto it, drizzle a little spit onto their head and allow a little incidental contact with your tongue or the side of your mouth. Let the moment linger before you close your mouth around them and give a long slow suck all the way from the base of their cock up to their head.

You Want Some of This?

08

Channel your inner exhibitionist while driving your partner mad for you by putting on a little show for them to remind them just how F-ing hot you are. Let them watch, but not touch, as you slowly smooth lube all over yourself. Drip a couple of dollops down your nipples, letting it linger for a moment, then slather it over your chest. Pour some onto your thighs, taking your time rubbing it in, gradually opening your legs. Drizzle some down your pussy or cock, and let them have a good long look. Don't let them touch you until you say so. See how desperate you can make them to get their hands on you. If you require begging, so be it.

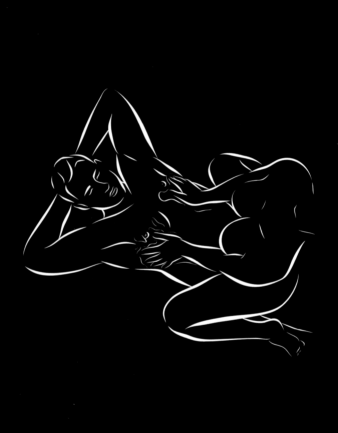

Lubey Love

09

Be super decadent and slather an obscene amount of lube all over them. Drip it on their thighs and belly and smear it around. Pour it on their chest, then lean over and rub it into them with your chest. Drizzle it on the head of their cock and watch it dribble down. Put on even more and stroke it over their balls and perineum. Oh, and put a blanket or a bunch of towels down first.

Show and Tell

10

Lube your hands up and ask your partner to put their hand over yours and show you how to stroke their penis. This is not being lazy! It's an actual hands-on masterclass on how they like to be touched. You'll gain all kinds of deep wisdom on the pressure and speed they use and what parts they focus on. Plus, it's superhot for them to feel your hands on them doing exactly what they like.

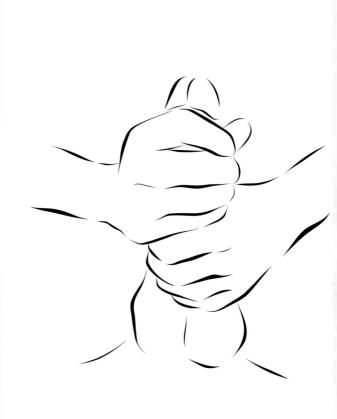

The Line Drive

Get them ready for more of you by using your finger to draw a wet line of lube from their butt hole to the tip of their penis. Draw lightly over their balls, then more on firmly on underside of shaft, especially on the base and frenulum. Retrace your path, using your tongue and a wet finger or fingers. Intensify the motion by gently cradling their balls and wrapping your hand around their shaft on the upstroke.

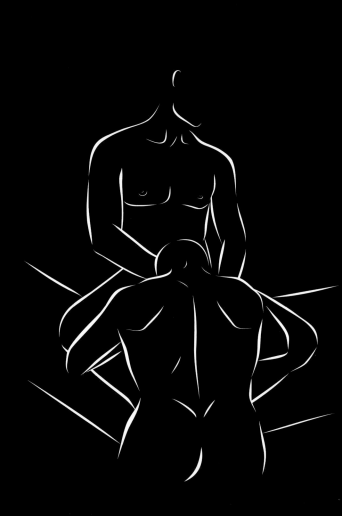

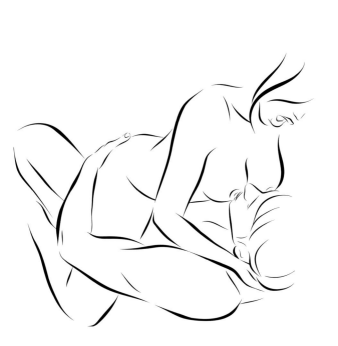

Slip 'N Slide

12

Lie your partner on their back then warm some lube between your hands and run your hands up their shaft, pressing their penis up against their belly. Slide some more warm lube up their shaft (why not?) then straddle them. Slide your lubey vulva or ass crack up and down their shaft, pressing against them. It's also an excellent option if your condoms have gone missing or if one or both among you don't want period sex.

Pretend I'm…

13

Give your partner the fantasy of being with another partner by blindfolding them and pretending to be someone else. Create a fantasy together with you as a celebrity, a made-up person, or someone you both know. Go all-in with your character. If they are a MILF, MILF it up. If they're a shy virgin, so are you. Just make sure that your character is someone you both agree on. And even though this is all completely pretend, it can be emotionally fraught, so make sure you're both up for it. If it gets too intense, either of you can stop it at any time—immediately, no questions asked. And debrief after, to reconnect and make sure you both get the reassurance you need.

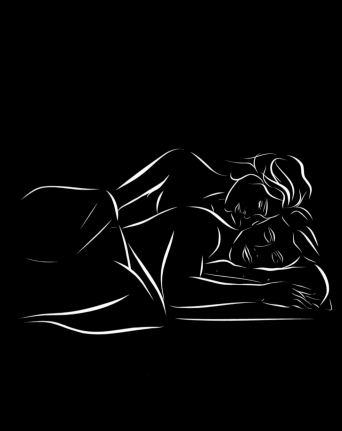

Story Time

14

Aural sex can be a surprisingly intimate way to create next-level heat with your partner. Lie next to them, with a lubed hand on their cock and your mouth next to their ear. As you stroke their cock, whisper things you know will drive them crazy. You can tell them how turned on you are touching them and how they feel in your hand or create a whole theater of the mind with a personalized fantasy.

Head Games

15

The head of the penis is super sensitive
and likes a lot of different kinds of
stimulation. Figure out which ones by
spending some focused time on just
the head. Some things to try: Swirl your
tongue around the head. Wrap your
lips around the rim, sucking gently
and turning your head back and forth.
Flick the frenulum with your tongue.
Pulse with your lips and tongue
around the ridge and head. Await
the forthcoming praise.

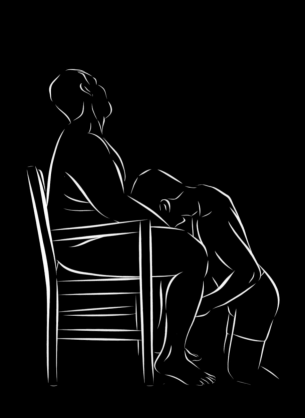

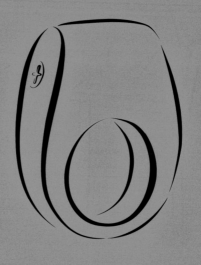

Magic Tongue

16

Zhuzh up a regular blow job with the help of a vibrating cock ring. Get a stretchy cock ring and put it around your tongue. Run your buzzing tongue up and down their shaft—use lube to smooth the way. Hover a bit on the frenulum, pressing your tongue firmly while wrapping your mouth around their head. If your partner is vibrator-averse, you can achieve a similar effect with just your mouth by making a buzzing sound.

Press and Play

Pressing their penis flat against your partner's belly not only makes them look huge(r), which is fun for all, but you can also use a lot of pressure for a firmer feel. Place your lubed, flat palms against the sides of their shaft and stroke up and down. You can stroke with your hands in unison or alternate. Enhance the sensations by using the bones in your palm to press against their cock for extra pressure.

The Up and Up

18

Create the feeling of an endless stroke by grasping the base of their penis with a lubed hand so that your thumb and index finger are pressed against your partner's abdomen. Squeeze tightly and pull their penis toward you, allowing your hand to roll over the tip. As your hand approaches the head, add the other hand at the base and pull up. Use firm pressure and a steady rhythm as you alternate your hands, maintaining constant contact.

Penis Sleeve Tease

19

Penis sleeves, a.k.a. male masturbators, are a kind of tube-shaped sex toy generally used for solo play, but there's no reason it can't work as a couples' toy. Surprise your partner by buying one for them and tell them they don't get to try it until later. That night (or whenever you decide they deserve it) make a big deal of getting it out of its packaging and talking about how you're gonna slide it over them. Make them wait for it to rev up their anticipation. Rub it across their mouth, trail it down their belly, press it next to their cock. Fill it with lube and let it drip onto their cock. Tease the head of their cock with one end of it, sliding it just a little bit on, before finally (!) sliding it down their entire shaft and letting it engulf them.

Play Ball

20

Balls are very sensitive, so be gentle when handling and always assess how it's going. Start by stroking them gently with your hands. Then try some of these techniques: Press your palm against the back of the balls, press them into your face, and draw a big slow W over the front side with hand or tongue. Flick the line that runs between them with your tongue or give it a slow luscious lick upwards. Take each one in your mouth and suck gently or swirl your tongue

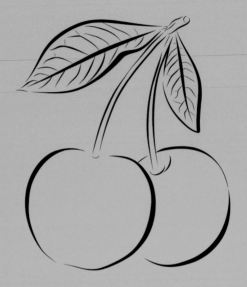

around one. Slather lube all over them and rub your face in them, exhaling so your partner can feel your warm breath. During a BJ, cup them with one warm hand and slowly pull them downward as you suck upward on their cock from base to tip.

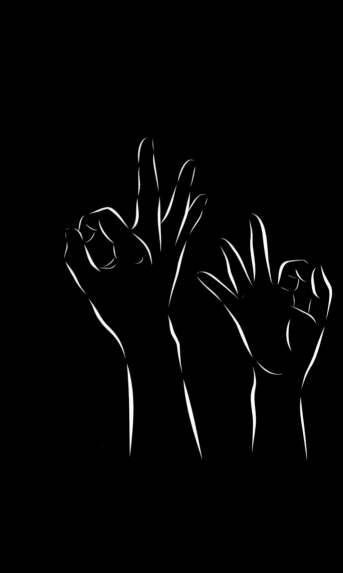

The Twister

21

Getting your hands involved can elevate a perfectly fine BJ into an incredible one. For this, make two okay signs with your lubed-up hands, then wrap your thumbs and forefingers around the base of their shaft. Sweep one hand up and over the head, with the other following behind. Add a twisting motion as you travel up their shaft. Or go from the middle of the shaft, one hand twisting up and the other down.

The Hummer

22

Add a whole bonus dimension to a blow job by using your mouth to create vibrations. Not only do the vibrations feel great (see also: the existence of vibrators), it's also just superhot to hear someone moaning for you. Start by pressing their penis up against their abdomen. Kneel by their side, running your mouth sideways up the bottom of their shaft, humming like you're playing a harmonica. Move your mouth up to suck on their head and then take their whole penis into your mouth, continuing to hum, then interspersing with moans. Go ahead and be loud. Let them hear through your moans just how much you like their cock. For extra points, fill your hand with lube and gently stroke their balls and/or press against their perineum.

Cock and Load

23

If your partner likes a tight grip, has a sensitive frenulum, and is already close to an orgasm, it is time to whip out the Cock and Load. Wrap both hands around the base of their lubed cock, interlacing your fingers on the upper side of their shaft. Point both thumbs upward toward the tip against the underside of their penis. Squeeze and stroke upward and trace small circles or hearts with your thumbs as they pass over the frenulum. You can use this to A. stoke their arousal even higher or B. take it all the way to an orgasm. If you both choose B. orgasm, maintain a tight, wet grip as you rub up and down at a rhythmic pace against their frenulum. Optional: Wear protective goggles, because there will be cum.

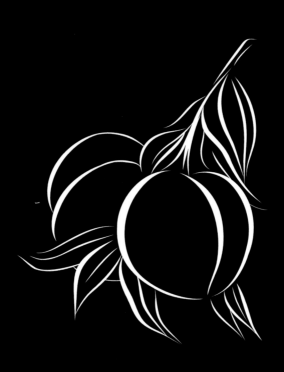

Bumhole Seduction

24

For any first foray into anal stuff, go slowly, use tons of lube and make sure your partner signs onto each new step. Start with anilingus, using your tongue to make circles around the butt hole and pressing your tongue gently into it. (If that's a little skeevy to you, try a dental dam.) If they are receptive, slowly slide a finger gently in. Stroke, tap, or just press firmly on the top wall of the anus.

The Lollipop

If they like a lot of extra attention to their head, give them the love they want by wrapping your lips around their head so that your mouth is on the rim. Make sure you cover your teeth with your lips because teeth = bad. Twist your head to the left and right make circles around the rim. Make it even freakier by flicking your tongue against their frenulum with heavy pressure as you twist.

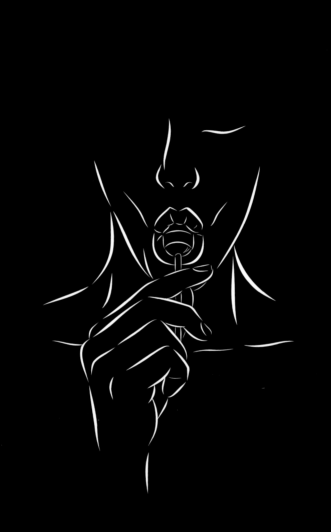

Instant Penis Ring

26

Cock rings have lots of benefits including stronger, more intense orgasms and keeping penises harder longer. But if your cock ring budget is tapped out, you can make one with your hands to get same benefits as the store-bought kind. Wrap your thumbs around the back of their balls and curl your index fingers around the base of their penis, creating a tight-ish circle. Keep your hands there as you suck on their balls, shaft, and head.

How Do You Like Me Now?

27

Get them ready for more of you by using your finger to draw a wet line of lube from their butt hole to the tip of their penis. Draw lightly over their balls, then more firmly on the underside of the shaft, especially on the base and frenulum. Retrace your path, using your tongue and a wet finger or fingers. Intensify the motion by gently cradling their balls and wrapping your hand around their shaft on the upstroke.

Grapefruiting

28

If you're in need of something a little extra to add to your repertoire, behold grapefruiting—using a hollowed out grapefruit as part of a vitamin C-fortified blow job. Start with a room temperature grapefruit. Roll it around to loosen the insides. Cut a penis-sized hole down the center. Slide the fruit over their penis and squeeze while you rub it up and down their shaft while sucking on their head.

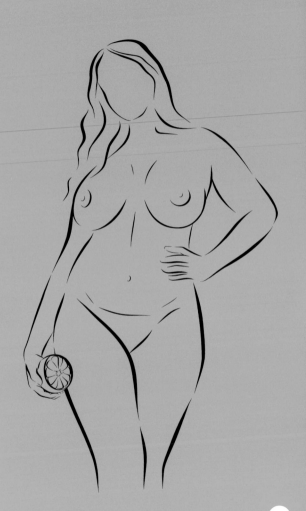

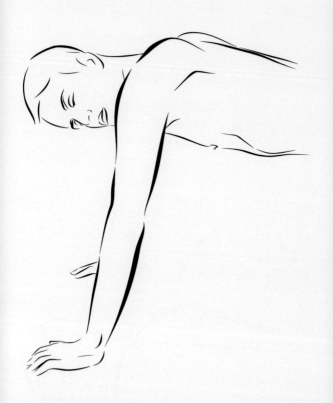

Woke Doggy

2 9

If they're up for some butt play (always ask first), have them get on their hands and knees à la doggy style. Kneel behind them and reach between their legs with a lubey hand and stroke their cock and balls until they're pressing their ass back for more. Drizzle some more lube down their ass crack, massaging it around the hole. Slide your finger inside as you stroke their cock. Sync your finger thrusts with your strokes.

Prostate Play

30

Knowing how to give someone a P-gasm is like having your own incredible superpower. P-gasms, or prostate orgasms, are stronger, more intense orgasms that can involve copious amounts of cum. They come from stimulating the prostate, a walnut-shaped gland a couple inches inside the rectum. To get to the spot, make sure your partner is well aroused with oral sex or a hand job. Once they're well-aroused, slide a lubed finger into their butt, feeling for a swollen area on the upper wall. Press, tap, or rub against it while one of your hands keeps stimulating their penis. Keep it up as they go through orgasm—it will enhance the sensations. If you don't want to put your finger in their butt and/or they want even stronger stimulation, you can also give the job to a P-spot toy, either vibrating or non-vibrating.